History Drawers On

History Drawers On

The Evolution of Women's Knickers

JACKIE STUART

AuthorHouse™
1663 Liberty Drive
Bloomington, IN 47403
www.authorhouse.com
Phone: 1-800-839-8640

First published by AuthorHouse   08/13/2011

ISBN: 978-1-4567-8967-1 (sc)
ISBN: 978-1-4567-8968-8 (ebk)

Printed in the United States of America

Contents

Foreword...vii

Chapter 1:   The Early Years 1795-1836............................ 1

Chapter 2:   The Victorian Years 1837-1901 9

Chapter 3:   The Early 20th Century 1902-1929............. 19

Chapter 4:   1930-1945: The Depression and

               World War II.. 34

Chapter 5:   Austerity to Affluence 1946-2010................. 50

Appendix 1: Time line.. 61

Appendix 2: Collecting drawers and knickers 63

INDEX 67

Foreword

Thomas Carlyle wrote in 1838 that the three great elements of modern civilization were Gunpowder, Printing, and the Protestant Religion. Another smaller, yet vital element he might have mentioned was the final adoption of hygienic washable underclothes, happening in his lifetime. To illustrate what mediaeval people did before this, (or rather did not do) there was a most famous late mediaeval manuscript illustration, the month of February from *Les Très Riches Heures du Duc de Berry*, painted about 1416. In the bottom left hand corner a peasant couple are shown warming themselves, their robes drawn up, in front of a large fire. Unlike the more demure young woman sitting near them, exposing at most only her calves and petticoat, the man and woman starkly reveal that they wore *nothing* beneath their garments. They were not alone, lords and ladies and the crowned heads of Europe wore nothing underneath either.

At some point, the idea of wearing linen drawers came to Northern Europe. Perhaps like gunpowder and printing mentioned above, it had an Eastern origin. The Turks of Central Asia and following them, the Ottoman Turks, had an insulting metaphor for poverty, vagabondage and lack of civilisation:—the word *donsuz*. It literally meant, and still means, 'without underpants.' The 13th century Mamluk warriors of Egypt, Kipchak Turks in origin, and trading partners with the Venetians, had as one of their heraldic emblems on their shields, the *sarawil al-futuwwa, i.e. the Trousers of Nobility.* They thought that only the very poor, savages, and infidels wore robes with nothing beneath. Perhaps because they were all descended from mounted warriors, they had discovered that trousers, drawers or underpants were most useful in the saddle.

How and why drawers came to Northern Europe, and why women there started wearing them, is not known for certain. However, in about 1667, Nell Gwyn is alleged in a satire to have appeared on stage wearing a newly fashionable pair of French drawers, apparently for display. This was for the delectation of the Restoration lechers in the audience, which might have included her future protector, His Majesty King Charles II. Respectable women then did not normally wear anything under their skirts, shifts and petticoats. Lady Mary Wortley Montagu, staying with her husband the ambassador in Istanbul in 1717-12, mentions putting on drawers [her word] as part of the outfit of a Turkish lady she was trying on. Yet it was not until the beginning of the 19th century that wearing drawers became common in England.

Thus in Britain from the beginning there was an uneasy association of what eventually became a useful and sometimes decorative item of clothing, with erotic significance and consequent taboos. This ambivalence has continued to the present day, and clouds the sober contemplation of what should have been a straightforward part of the history of textiles and dress. The social taboos were so strong that now it is not easy to find good illustrations, examples or even descriptions, of these historic garments before the very late 19th century. Added to this difficulty are the constantly changing names and styles for these garments. Since the beginning of the 19th century up to the present day, they have been called, amongst a host of coy euphemisms, *drawers, knickerbockers, pantalettes, pantaloons, bloomers, combinations, lingerie, pants, smalls, briefs, panties, knickers, thongs*. Worse still, some of these names, depending on date and context, mean quite different things. For example *bloomers* could mean either the Turkish-style trousers for women's outerwear, underneath a short skirt, advocated by Mrs Bloomer the American in the 1860s; or subsequently, large drawers used for underwear in the late 19th and 20th centuries. *Knickers* or *knickerbockers* as terms have an even more complex origin and history of use, and even now mean different things to British and American audiences.

In the present day, although most taboos have allegedly disappeared, there is still some conflict between the [mostly male] erotic idea that underwear enhances the female body, and the intermittent female ambivalence about the consequences of this. People still feel uncomfortable about *intimate* garments, and so discussion of them for some people is a social taboo still. So paradoxical are the ways of fashion that for a long time wearing closed drawers was actually regarded as a bad and unhealthy thing, as opposed to wearing open ones or none at all; yet in the 20th century the reverse became true. So at one time wearing drawers [like Nell above] was indicative of depravity, but in the modern era, the saying in Britain:—'wearing a fur coat [or red hat] *and no knickers*' was a coarse and deliberate insult.

In this book you will find a sober and dispassionate chronological history, with copious illustrations, descriptions and quotations from people who saw them, made them, wore them, (or chose not to.) Given that virtually all women now wear knickers of one form or another, it does seem strange

Jackie Stuart

that there are so few texts that have dealt with the subject, especially with what the majority of people wore. So, here at last is an illustrated survey of the last 340 years of the twists and turns of fashion in the hitherto mysterious underworld of historic knickers.

Charles Newton. A Former Curator at the Victoria & Albert Museum

Chapter 1

The Early Years 1795-1836

According to James Laver, who was a costume historian and a curator at the Victoria and Albert Museum in the mid 20th century, 'The earlier part of the history of underclothes is obscure by reason of its very simplicity, for there were really no underclothes as we know them.' (1)

Many people are surprised to learn that the history of drawers for British women dates back only to the late 18th century. Prior to this it seems they wore only underskirts and stockings beneath the lower half of their dresses. It is startling to imagine that Queen Elizabeth I, who reigned 1558-1603, would not have worn drawers beneath the raiment that we see in her portraits, although we know she wore knitted silk stockings secured with a garter.

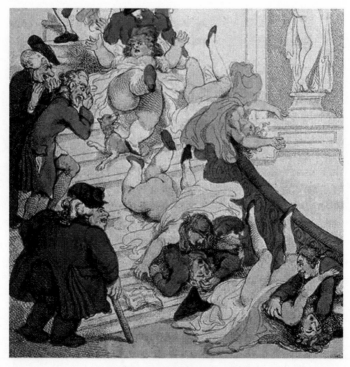

Thomas Rowlandson cartoon
'The Stare Case' c. 1800

The very early history of underwear is particularly sketchy. Some of the first known knicker-like garments can be seen in the Louvre on a Sumerian terracotta and bas relief dating from 3000 BC. These are very skimpy and surprisingly similar to modern briefs in form if not in function; they are evidently outer garments rather than underwear. The same is true of the bikini-like apparel sported by female athletes in certain Roman mosaics from the 4th century AD. Back in the Dark Ages, British women are known to have worn a type of dress like a fabric wrap but there is no evidence about whether they wore anything beneath this. Early historical written documents about life in Britain provide scant details about clothing of any kind and although paintings and sculptures provide good evidence of outer wear the majority do not privilege the viewer to know what their subjects wore beneath (though one exception is the medieval image described in the Foreword to this book).

Drawers are known to have been worn by Catherine de Medici (1519-1589), a Florentine socialite who married into the French Royal Family and became Queen Consort of France. She introduced drawers to the French aristocracy who apparently wore them mainly for horse riding (2). Writing in the 17th century, Samuel Pepys made a reference to his wife's drawers in his diary, but as she was French, she would have brought this fashion with her to Britain from France.

Historically speaking most new fashions in Britain, including underwear, have first been worn by the aristocracy and then some of them gradually filtered down through the different levels of society. This process often took some time. When upper class women began to wear drawers in the early 19th century, it was seventy years or more before the trend was picked up by the working class. As fashions changed, older women often rejected the new styles and continued to wear fashions from their younger years. This can be seen in photographs of the British Royal Family of the 1920s where the younger women are dressed in trendy clothes whilst Queen Mary is wearing styles some twenty years out of date. The same attitudes were apparent with underwear, resulting in a range of styles of drawers being worn by women of different generations.

There is evidence from my own collection that some drawers have been altered over the years to conform to changes in fashion or the personal needs of the wearer. For example, some were made entirely by hand, but have small areas sewn by machine, which indicates that alterations were made many years later.

The terms used to describe drawers have varied enormously according to the class and age of the women who wore them, as well as the geographical location. Country women would have worn more old-fashioned drawers than those who lived in the towns. Over the last two hundred years, underwear for the lower body worn by British women has been variously been known as pantaloons, pantalettes, drawers, bloomers, knickers, panties, trunks and briefs. The reason that we still refer to our modern knickers as 'a pair' even though they are a single item harks back to the days when they were a garment of two separate halves held together at the waist (see below for more details).

Underwear styles have always been influenced by dress fashions and by social and economic issues such as wars and recessions. Other important changes have resulted from the invention of new fabrics such as rayon and nylon and this book will explore the ramifications of these innovations in detail.

The first leg coverings worn as underwear by British women date from the late 18th century. During the Directory Period in France (1795-1799) some French women wore flesh-coloured underwear beneath the diaphanous muslin dresses that were fashionable at the time so that they appeared to be otherwise naked (3). This idea appears to have been adopted by some young British women who wore long-legged, closed-crotch

4

underwear which had been invented for theatrical wear by the Frenchman Jean-Christophe Maillot who was a costumier for the Opera de Paris in the late 18th century. These garments were called pantaloons after the men's leg-hugging trousers from which they evolved, but the term was soon feminised to pantalettes and an open-crotch design quickly became popular. Some young women wore pantaloons (or pantalettes) to below their dress hem with a frill around the lower edges so that the trimming could be displayed.

The wearing of closed-crotch pantaloons by women in Britain was very short lived as these were seen as unfeminine and indecent and too similar to trousers worn by men. This was a problem as the Bible states that 'the woman shall not wear that which pertaineth unto a man . . . for all that do so are an abomination to the Lord their God' (Deuteronomy, Chapter 22, verse 5). When Joan of Arc was tried for witchcraft in the 14th century her accusers made ammunition of the fact that she wore men's clothes.

In the early 19th century, drawers were worn by women that consisted of two tubes of fabric covering the legs and the outside of the hips, tied together with tape around the waist. They were quite plain in design and this open-crotch design was considered to be less masculine, so less sinful and therefore much more acceptable. All drawers at this time were hand-made either by dressmakers or seamstresses as the sewing machine had not yet been invented. The styles were almost certainly adapted according to the wearer's needs and wishes. The early history of pantaloons and drawers is not very well documented and costume historians have slightly differing views on exactly what was worn and accepted when. For example, Pearl Binder, author of *Muffs and Morals*, wrote that as drawers in this period were considered by many to be 'depraved, unnatural and vicious' (4) they were simply not discussed or written about at the time. James Laver claimed that in the late 1790s 'some women wore complete outfits of tights, sometimes white, sometimes flesh coloured'. (5) Unfortunately, neither of these very good costume historians provided a reference for these statements, so their sources for this information remain unknown.

The History of Underclothes by C. Willett Cunnington and Phillis Cunnington quoted from a letter written by Lady Stanley in 1801 in which she described a woman who was 'lately walking about Brighton in a muslin gown over a pair of grey pantaloons tied at the ankle with black twist'. She went on to assert that this was a 'masculine style of wear'. (6) The Cunningtons also quote from an article in *The Times* (1798) which mentioned a lady at a ball in Dublin who was wearing 'flesh coloured pantaloons over which was a gauze petticoat'. Both sides of the petticoat were apparently tucked up over her hips to show her thighs. The Cunningtons provided pictures of early open-crotch drawers: a pair in knitted silk dated 1810-20 and a pair of lawn drawers worn by the Duchess of Kent in 1820. (7) Most drawers at this time were made of cotton or linen.

In 1811 Lady de Clifford was visiting the 15-year-old Princess Charlotte (the only child of the Prince Regent) who was sitting with her legs stretched out and showing her drawers. Lady de Clifford complained to her that they were 'too long'. The Princess replied: 'I do not think so. The Duchess of Bedford's are much longer, and they are edged by Brussels lace'. (8) This suggests that drawers were being worn by royalty and the aristocracy at this time.

Around 1820 it seems that drawers became shorter and by 1830 they were no longer an important fashion item for older women. It is likely that they were still being worn by a few aristocratic women for horse riding and some special occasions. However, they were certainly still worn by little girls who wore shorter dresses, as is shown by many photographs of the period. These children's drawers continued to be known as pantalettes, although some consisted of two completely separate tubes covering the legs which were tied individually above the knee.

Old drawers kept by museums and collectors are not always possible to date accurately unless the provenance is known or if they were part of a known *trousseau* (a set of garments for a honeymoon). As advertisements are a late 19th century innovation they cannot, unfortunately, be enlisted to help date older styles. Advertising in its modern form is much more helpful to the costume historian as demonstrated in later chapters of this book.

Chapter 1 references

1. Laver J, *Taste and Fashion from the French Revolution to the Present Day*, 1945, p.136
2. Saint-Laurent C and Norman J, *The History of Ladies Underwear*, 1966, p.84
3. Laver J, *Taste and Fashion from the French Revolution to the Present Day*, 1945, p.137
4. Binder P, *Muffs and Morals: An Account of Dress and Fashion in Relation to Moral Standards*, 1953, p.24
5. Laver J, *Taste and Fashion from the French Revolution to the Present Day*, 1945, p.137

6. Willett Cunnington C and Cunnington P, *The History of Underclothes,*1951, p.108
7. Willett Cunnington C and Cunnington P, *The History of Underclothes,*1951, p.113
8. Ewing E, *Dress and Undress: A History of Women's Underwear*, 1978, p.56

Chapter 2

THE VICTORIAN YEARS 1837-1901

Following a dip in popularity in the 1830s, where the reasons are not clear, drawers came back into fashion in the 1840s. Drawers remained quite plain at this time and according to *The Handbook of the Toilet* in 1841, ladies drawers at the time could be made of flannel, angola, calico (a cheap plain weave cotton), cotton stocking-web' (machine knitted fabric), longcloth (a closely woven cotton), as well as chamois leather for riding'. (1) Many people believe that the word angola is the wrong term for angora, but the Angora goat produced mohair which would have been much too itchy for underwear, and the Angora rabbit hair was not made into a fabric at that time. The Girls Home Companion, a book published in 1881, noted clothing being made from Angola cotton, so it is likely that the word angola meant a form of cotton. Throughout the 19th century the popular length for drawers changed many times, rising and falling as fashion.

The 1850s saw the introduction of hooped petticoats made from crinoline, which was originally a stiff horse-hair fabric that had been used earlier in the century. The 'crinoline' petticoats in the latter half of the century were no longer made of crinoline but were still referred to by this name. They were supported by hoops of whalebone, or (later) steel, which held the skirts of dresses well away from the legs. This meant that when women bent over or climbed a step the lower half of their legs would show. If they fell over, of course, then a lot more besides may have been inadvertently put on display! This promoted the wearing of much longer and more ornate drawers that would cover the whole length of the leg and also be decorative. It soon became much more acceptable for drawers to show beneath the dress hems, although they continued to be of open crotch design. White embroidery and Broderie Anglaise, which consisted of a scalloped buttonhole edging with designs made from ovals and triangles, were very popular at this time. Crinolines were only worn by upper- and middle-class women.

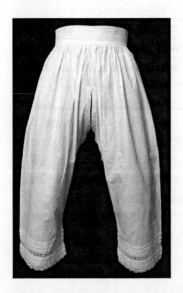

White handmade drawers with hand sewn Broderie Anglaise. The pintucks are machine sewn, so this was possibly a method of shortening them many years later and not needing to remove the embroidery. c.1850 Author's collection.

Drawers were still clearly a taboo subject, as noted by Lady Chesterfield in a letter she wrote in 1850 stating that drawers were 'comfortable garments we all wear but none of us talk about'. (2) It was another ten years before drawers became socially acceptable to be worn by middle-class women, but affordability was also an issue. In 1851, the Singer Sewing Machine was invented but the high cost of the first models ensured that they were available only to the wealthy for the use of their dressmakers.

In the next decade, quite a few drawers were ready-made and available to buy in shops. Some were still made by dressmakers and sewn by hand, while others were machine-made. In 1867, Chas Ammot & Co. of St Paul's Churchyard announced in the *Illustrated London News* that they were selling 'tucked drawers' which were a popular fashion of the time.(3) Tucks were similar to pleats, but were horizontal rather than vertical. Tucks had been hand made earlier, but once the sewing machine was used, it would have been much easier to make tucks.

In the 1860s, middle-class women began to wear drawers made from flannel and knitted cotton during the winter, and fine woven linen or cotton drawers during the warmer seasons. Frills became popular due to the invention of the sewing machine which made them much easier to apply. Many drawers appear to have been knee length at this time, although it is likely that older styles were still being worn.

In 1860, Mrs Amelia Bloomer, an American women's dress reformer, advocated the use of a type of trousers for women to wear under a knee-length skirt which became known as 'bloomers'. They were wide, full-length trousers gathered at the ankle and of a Turkish style. This fashion never caught on seriously in Britain, but a bloomer style of trousers was used by some women later in the century for cycling. Some drawers in Britain were now referred to as bloomers, although the original garment was outerwear.

In 1869, the Butterick pattern company produced patterns for drawers and ladies knickerbockers. Prior to this time dressmakers would have made drawers to fit their customers without the use of a company-produced paper pattern. These drawers made by dressmakers might have conformed to a current fashion, but would also have allowed changes to the design as required by the customer for longer and shorter legs, or different styles of embroidery or lace. The Butterick pattern for drawers also suggested making them with scarlet flannel which was clearly an acceptable fabric at the time.

Crinoline petticoats were still being worn by wealthy and upper-class women, as noted by Lady Eleanor Stanley in her diary when she referred to the Duchess of Manchester who fell when climbing over a stile: 'a part of her underclothing consisted of a pair of scarlet tartan knickerbockers (the things Charlie shoots in)'.(4)

Knickerbockers were originally an item of men's outerwear that were loose fitting and gathered below the knee. They were worn for sport and leisure. A man who wrote The History of New York early in the 19th Century, used the pseudonym of Dietrich Knickerbocker and as he was very keen on sport, it is likely that this style of trousers was named after him as he would have worn then. From the 1860s onwards there are references to knickerbockers worn by women, and no pictures or details of their design are forthcoming, although the Cunningtons suggested that towards the end of the century they 'were made with a buttoned flap at the back' rather than being gusset free.(5)

When Prince Albert, Consort of Queen Victoria, died in 1867, black mourning clothes became very fashionable for those who were grieving for a deceased family member. As most drawers at this time were white, and others in pastel colours, some women slotted black ribbon through the hems to make them more in keeping with their black mourning dresses and coats.

The 1870s saw the end of the crinoline when dresses became much tighter fitting around the lower half of the body with a bustle (a gathering of fabric) at the back. This meant that when women bent over their ankles were not so readily on display. Most drawers now finished at the knee and were edged with a frill. By this time a few drawers were being worn with a closed crotch and some women referred to these as 'knickers'. They often had buttons at the side of the waist and some were made of silk for use by well-off women.

> "When I was a child I wore long-legged, open-gusset combinations which my mother made, but when I became a kitchen maid in the 1890s, I made much shorter ones, but with an open crotch. I remember using calico." (1958)
>
> Mary Curtis, born 1877.

Some working-class women had only just begun to wear open-crotch drawers by the 1880s, whilst the closed-crotch style was beginning to find favour with the upper classes. Working-class women usually hand-sewed their own drawers and made them from cheap fabrics such as calico or cotton longcloth. Many of these garments have survived and are available to collectors. It was standard practice for working-class women to be given used clothes by their employers and this would have included drawers. Second-hand clothing was often sold on street markets and would have made drawers available to the working classes.

Towards the end of the decade, the Princess Line became popular. This was a fashion promoted by Princess Alexandra where the skirt and bodice of a dress were not made separately, as they had been in the past. For this style, seams ran vertically from the shoulder down to the thighs or even further, rather than around the waist or under the bust. It provided quite a smooth line, so some changes needed to be made to underwear so that they did not show beneath the waist. Combinations, which spliced the chemise (an undergarment similar to a modern knee-length petticoat) and drawers, were introduced and often followed the Princess Line pattern, having no seam around the waist. The early ones had quite long legs and continued to be highly decorated with open-work embroidery such as Broderie Anglaise and lace. White embroidered feather stitching was also very popular around this time for all underwear. In 1897, the *Lady's Realm* magazine noted: 'The fashion for wearing combinations is followed by very few people and indeed, one may say, by none of the smart set, who never really took to this form of underwear.' (6)

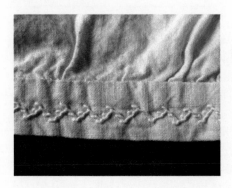

Feather stitch around the hem of white cotton drawers. c. 1880s. Author's collection.

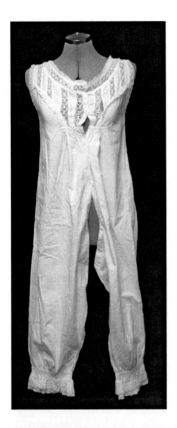

White cotton combinations worn under Princess Line with open crotch. c.1880 Author's collection

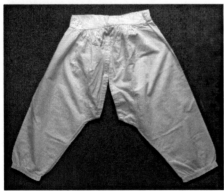

Cream calico open crotch drawers edged with feather stitch. c.1890 Author's collection

Health as well as fashion was a consideration for women when choosing underwear. Some women believed vehemently that health and comfort were more important than fashion or social convention in making such choices. The Rational Dress Society was founded in London in 1881. Its members protested against clothes that deformed the body, causing difficulties in bodily movement, and any form of clothing that might damage a woman's health. They did not approve of tight corsets, or high-heeled shoes. In 1884 they promoted the idea of a divided skirt under a long coat, which would enable women to move freely and exercise. Cycling was now a popular pastime for many women, so they sometimes wore a divided skirt such as this, or bloomer style trousers under an ordinary skirt. Both were seen by many women as provocative, so most women continued to cycle in long skirts worn with drawers or knickers.

For health reasons, Dr Gustav Jaeger, a German zoologist, advocated the wearing of animal fibres next to the skin, rather than those derived from plants, as these allowed 'noxious exhalations' to leave the body, making them healthier to wear. The theory gained currency and was even supported in an 1884 edition of *The Lancet*, the top medical journal. Consequently woollen underwear soon became fashionable for use in cold weather. Jaeger combinations and drawers were made in stockinette with buttons to the front, and cuffs at the wrists and ankles. Jaeger clothing has changed considerably over time but the company is still producing high quality garments in a range of fibres, including synthetic ones.

Aertex, a loosely woven cotton cellular fabric which was promoted as soft, comfortable and hygienic, was invented in 1888. At first it was only used for making men's underwear, but by the early 1890s the Aertex Company expanded their operations into the manufacture of ladies' combinations which were similar in style to those made by Jaeger. This fabric remained very popular throughout the first half of the 20th century and continues to be used for some menswear, sports wear and women's underwear today.

The first advertisements for underwear began in the 1890s. Naturally, advertisements offer valuable assistance to the costume historian, although earlier examples of adverts often shy away from depicting the garments clearly and show them folded rather than being worn by a model. As noted earlier, the fashion for the length of drawers varied widely throughout the 19th century, but in 1895, drawers were mainly ending at the knee in a gathered style, though some styles were loose and open at the knee.

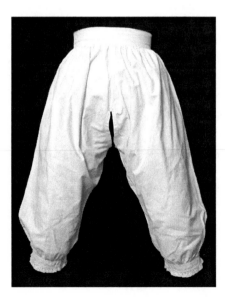

White cotton open crotch drawers handmade. c.1890 Author's collection.

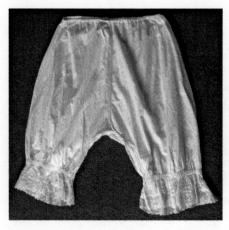

Closed crotch
white cotton lawn
knickers machine
made. c.1900.
Author's collection.

Chapter 2 references

1   Willett Cunnington C and Cunnington P, *The History of Underclothes,*1951, p.148
2   Binder P, *Muffs and Morals: An Account of Dress and Fashion in Relation to Moral Standards*, 1953, p.24
3   *Shops and Shopping 1800-1914 (Where, and in What Manner the Well-Dressed Englishwoman Bought Her clothes)* by Alison Adburgham, 1967, p.130
4   Willett Cunnington C and Cunnington P, *The History of Underclothes,*1951, p.155
5   Willett Cunnington C and Cunnington P, *The History of Underclothes,*1951, p.196
6   Ewing E, *Dress and Undress: A History of Women's Underwear*, 1978, p.91

Chapter 3

THE EARLY 20TH CENTURY

1902-1929

In the early 1900s, dress fashions became very frilly and adorned with lace and embroidery. This popular style of clothing also included underwear which was now referred to as lingerie (from the French word for underwear). Closed crotch drawers became more acceptable and by 1910 they were widely available, although working and older women still preferred to wear drawers with an open crotch and most continued to make their own. The word 'drawers' was still used by many women whether or not the crotch was open or closed.

"When I was a kitchen maid in the 1890s I only wore open drawers. They were also what my friends and family wore. Open drawers were seen as more hygienic. I made them myself from calico, but also made some flannel ones for the winter. Those who wore closed drawers would have had to wash them more often." (1958)
Mary Curtis, born 1877.

The wearing of closed drawers towards the end of the 19th century could be attributed to the new found confidence and independence of upper- and middle-class women. This change in women's status gave rise to the term the 'New Woman'. More women were receiving a higher education, enabling them to become employed in professional jobs. Manchester University began to offer degrees for women in 1880 and in 1900 there were 200 qualified women doctors in Britain. However, it was not until 1910 that women could become barristers and bankers. Women were now determined to obtain the right to vote. Their campaign was successful in 1919 for women aged over 30, and then in 1928 all British women were granted the same voting rights as men. These profound social changes allowed women to ignore the perceived prohibition on 'dressing as men' (i.e. wearing closed-crotch drawers) and to wear what was comfortable and appropriate to their altered circumstances. This 'New Woman' also enjoyed sporting activities such as tennis, golf, ice-skating and riding bicycles. All these sports would clearly have necessitated the wearing of closed-crotch drawers.

The hems of drawers continued to be ornate and Madeira embroidery was very popular from around 1905 and was much used. This consisted of patterns made in fine buttonhole stitching and dots. Embroidered monograms on underwear were also popular. From about 1906 underwear was routinely trimmed with baby ribbon. The hems around the legs of drawers were adorned with lace or embroidery that had holes or slits that would allow ribbon to be threaded through.

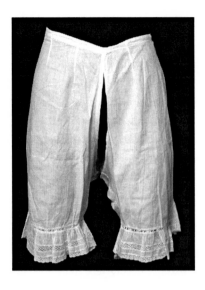

Early 20th century
open crotch white
drawers with broken
yellow silk ribbon
threaded through
the knee area.
Author's collection.

In 1906, Butterick produced a pattern for 'French Open Drawers' with a frill around the legs (pattern number 9495). They were very wide and knee length and this was a style that remained fashionable until the 1920s.

> My mother told me that in 1905 her sister
> returned home from her honeymoon and invited
> her upstairs to see the 'latest thing in underwear'.
> She showed her three pairs of nainsook
> combinations which had elastic around the legs
> and closed gussets. Her sister said, 'I will cut the
> gussets out because they're not healthy'. (2009)
> Ruby Fisher, Milliner, born 1913.

In *The Manual of Needlework and Cutting Out* of 1907 (1) there were patterns for drawers and knickerbockers. For the drawers, it suggests that the length from waist to the leg hem should be between 16 and 32 inches; the longer of these almost reaching the ankle whilst the shorter one is halfway down the thigh which seems quite short for the time. It says that the 'width of leg at the knee' should be '2/3 or 5/8 of the whole width of the leg' and describes a waistband and side openings. This book was written for teachers of sewing, and did not give details of whether or not the crotch of the drawers should be sewn together as the teachers could decide that for themselves. The same book had a pattern for knickerbockers with a waistband and leg bands rather than elastic. Both styles suggest using bleached or unbleached calico or flannelette. The knickerbockers would be more likely to have a closed crotch, but women who made their own underclothes were able to adapt them to an open crotch style if they wished. The same book provided details of how to do feather stitching, which was still a very popular embroidery stitch for underwear at that time.

In 1907, the same year that the book referenced above was published, The Army and Navy Stores were advertising underclothes that were machine, or hand-made. The hand-made ones were more expensive. This shows that times had changed and underwear was now being factory-made on machines, which made it more affordable than clothing made by dressmakers using traditional hand-sewing techniques. Many women still made their own underwear, but buying machine-made garments was becoming more and more common.

Directoire knickers were first worn around 1908, and were designed for wearing with the popular new Directoire style of dresses created by French fashion designer Paul Poiret (who was inspired by the fashions of the Directory Period in France around 1800). The early Directoire knickers were a style that came to below the knee and were gathered into a binding strip using the same fabric. It seems that they rose above the knee during the next decade and were a very acceptable type of closed-crotch knickers, which were being made in several different colours. Some were beginning to have elastic around the waist and legs. The term knickerbocker was now used for a directoire style that had a flap at the back.

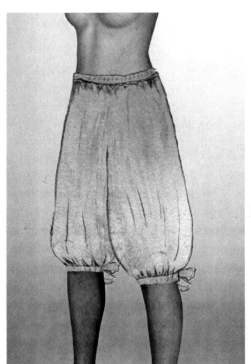

Directoire knickers as sold by Gamages in 1914

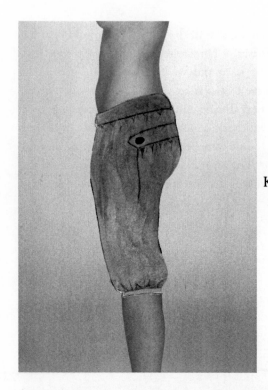

Knickerbockers
as sold by
Gamages in
1914

Jill Fields, Professor of History at California State University, Fresno, noted in her book *An Intimate Affair* (2) that the very popular Tango dance began in the USA in 1911 and moved to Great Britain a couple of years later, and this had a significant impact on underwear fashions. She refers to the Cunningtons who state in their book *The History of Underclothes* that in 1914 'Tango knickers were advertised' and were known to have a closed crotch. Tango knickers were described by the Cunningtons as 'one length of material falling from the waist in front to the knees and up again to the waist at the back, with slits at the sides for the legs.' It is difficult to know how widely used these were because there are few references to them and no records of them being in museum collections.

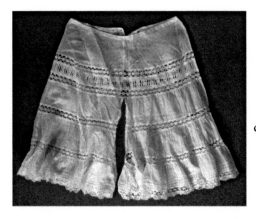

White skirt
knickers with
open crotch.
c.1910 Author's
coon

Around 2010 some knickers became shorter, much wider and fancier and they were known as skirt knickers.

A catalogue from Gamages (a London department store) in 1914 advertised knickers in 'trimmed longcloth', a closely woven cotton fabric which was produced in long lengths, and 'nainsook', a loosely woven cotton fabric. Some of the items in this catalogue were 'trimmed with Swiss embroidery of good design' and ribbons. Also on offer were 'Peg-top-skirt knickers in mercerised sateen with frill; Colours: white, pink, saxe, cream, silvery grey, heliotan, navy and black'. Peg-top dresses were in high fashion at this time; these were fairly tight and straight reaching the ankles, but they had an overskirt which was hitched up onto the hips. The peg-top knickers were around knee length with a frill and were pulled up at the side over each thigh, sometimes secured with ribbon or a rosette.

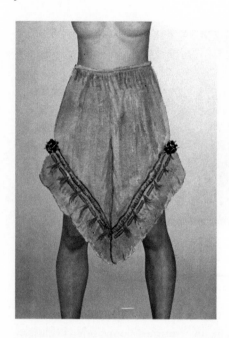

Peg top knickers
as sold by
Gamages in 1914

In 1916, a Butterick guide for dressmakers assumed a preference for open-crotch knickers as it produced only brief instructions for closed ones. This indicates that that there were still many women who did not wish to wear knickers with a closed crotch. However, this may principally have been a preference among women who made their own drawers because of an aversion to the closed-crotch alternatives.

With the First World War (1914-18) came a period of profound social upheaval. As the nation's menfolk were called away to fight in the trenches, women were obliged to take on their temporarily-vacated civilian jobs or to work on the land or in the munitions factories. Naturally women in these positions quickly forsook their impractical skirts and dresses in favour of trousers and this in turn promoted the wearing of closed drawers for reasons of comfort and hygiene.

Some black underwear was worn during this time, probably under black dresses. However, it was not wholly acceptable to most women for general wear as it was seen as erotic. The *Vogue* magazine advertised some cami-knickers in 1916 that were red with black frills around the legs and the top. The same magazine also advertised black cami-knickers in 1924. Cami-knickers consisted of a camisole and knickers made in one piece. The camisole was an item of underwear which covered the upper body to the waist.

Chemi-knickers, which consisted of a chemise with a button underneath, were introduced around 1917. They were also called step-ins and cami-combinations, but the Americans called them 'envelope chemises'. A chemise was an undergarment similar to a modern knee-length petticoat. The old-style combinations started to disappear and newer combinations became shorter in the leg and much fancier than their predecessors.

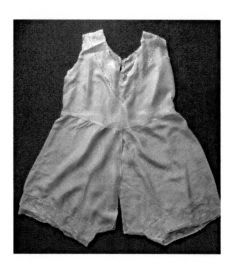

Very fine pink silk open crotch combinations c. 1918. Author's collection.

The mid-1920s saw the shortest skirts ever known up to that time, ending just above the knee, which dictated the wearing of closed-crotch knickers that were shorter than those worn previously. This was a decade of great social pleasure with many parties, dances and fun times available made possible by an improvement in the country's economy. Young people enjoyed learning the new dances from the USA such as The Charleston and The Black Bottom, both of which involved moving fast and jumping around. The short dresses worn by young women would have flipped around, often showing their thighs and underwear. In her autobiography, the Duchess of Argyle noted that when she was a young woman in the 1920s her mother made a comment having heard that her daughter planned to attend a dance one evening: 'If you are going to be flung around the ballroom by Billy, I insist that nanny buys you a pair of bloomers with elastic round the legs.' (3)

French knickers became fashionable in the later part of the decade with wide, square legs ending at the knee and often featuring ornate embroidery. However, Directoire knickers were still considered to be practical. Almost all fashionable knickers now had a closed crotch, though many older women continued to wear open-crotch drawers.

Cami-knickers grew in popularity in the 1920s, particularly those made from Crepe de Chine, as silk fabrics were now much more available than during the years of the war. They fitted very nicely underneath the skimpy dresses of the time and were very light to wear. Lingerie at this time was narrow and not bulky.

During this era, many different styles of knickers were being worn. Cami-knickers could have been loose or tight around the legs and some still had an open crotch. Cami-bockers were introduced, which were like cami-knickers but elasticated around the legs just above the knee and with a buttoned opening at the back. Some knickers were very frilly and lacy, while others were embroidered or adorned with ribbon. By now lingerie was also being referred to as 'undies'.

In 1928, the Sartor Manufacturing Company produced a mail order catalogue which demonstrated the fashionable wear of the time. It contained mostly Directoire-style knickers, with cami-bockers noted as 'a new style garment'. It also included tight-fitting combinations which were referred as 'combs'. Interestingly no French knickers were shown, perhaps because French knickers were worn by middle- and upper-class wealthy women at this time and the catalogue was probably designed to sell to the lower classes.

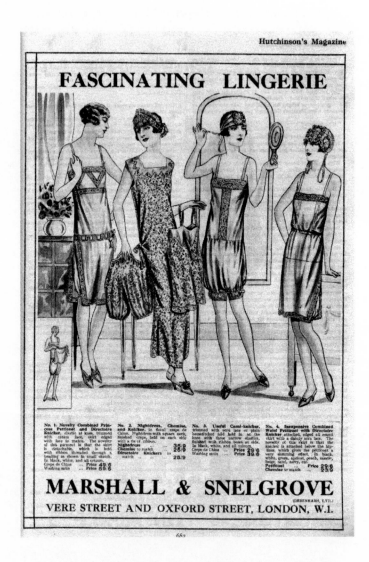

Advertisement from Hutchinson's Magazine October 1927

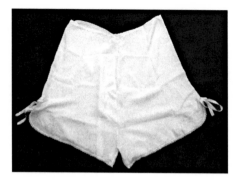

Hand sewn and
embroidered
cream silk
French knickers
c.1930 Author's
collection

I never wore French knickers as a young
woman or even when more mature
because they were always too expensive.
(2009)

Phyllis Dyke, Nurse, born 1925.

The undergarments in the 1928 Sartor catalogue were all
made from rayon fabrics. Although cellulose fibres (such as
rayon) were invented in 1884 by the French chemist Amselme
Payen, it was not until the late 1920s that they began to be
used for clothing and underwear. In 1925 the Federal Trade
Commission in the USA permitted the use of the name
'Rayon' for cellulose fabrics.

The fact that there are no French knickers in rayon from this
period could be attributable to problems with the quality of
the cellulose fibres, which may not have been fine enough
for this delicate style. However, pure silk underwear was
prohibitively expensive. In his book *20th Century Fashion*,
John Peacock shows very detailed pictures of clothes from top

international designers of the 1920s, including French knickers and cami-knickers which he said were made from silk—these items were only worn by the upper echelons of society. (4)

In 1928, the 'trinity set' emerged, which consisted of a chemise top, a petticoat to the knees and Directoire knickers—all three garments made into one. Some were made of very practical fabrics such as locknit (or knitted rayon: a popular, hard-wearing fabric), but others were made from superb delicate silk fabrics. Rayon in the 1920s was not a fabric that had a good reputation, but the quality was improving all the time, as will be seen in the next chapter.

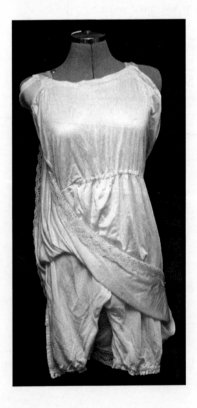

Cream rayon locknit
Trinity Set 1928
Author's collection.

Chapter 3 references

1   Walker A, *The Manual of Needlework and Cutting Out: Specially Adapted for Teachers of Sewing, Students and Pupil Teachers*, 1907
2   Jill Fields, *An Intimate Affair: Women, Lingerie and Sexuality*, 2007, p.32
3   Campbell M (Duchess of Argyll), *Forget Not*, 1977
4   Peacock J, *20th Century Fashion: The Complete Sourcebook*, 1993

Chapter 4

1930-1945: The Depression and World War II

During the 1930s, the optimism and devil-may-care spirit of the 1920s receded in the face of the Great Depression and the growing threat of another war in Europe. The Depression years also created a decline in consumer purchasing-power. Despite the privations and uncertainties of the time, the innovations of fashion designers continued apace.

In the early 1930s dress styles became longer and more feminine. French fashion designer Madeleine Vionnet designed a style of dress that was bias cut and slim-fitting. Bias cutting, also known as cutting on the cross, meant placing the pattern diagonally onto the fabric so that the garment would cling tightly to the body with the stretch going vertically and horizontally. This design was quickly adopted throughout Europe and the USA and soon became the height of fashion.

Due to the clinging styles of these new fashions, which were often made of smooth shiny fabrics, underwear needed to be very discreet so that seams and folds did not show through the dresses. Of course, not all women wore this style of costume, but like most popular fashions it was generally worn for weddings, parties, dances and most social events. The best fabric to wear under these tight-fitting dresses was silk, as it is very fine and light and would not show any creases, but of course this was an expensive luxury item and consequently not an option for everyone. Rayon, the cheaper manufactured fabric was pressed into service as a substitute, as was fine, soft cotton.

Many dresses for daytime wear that were sold in shops were similar in style and bias cut, but there were always women who made their own clothes in a design that was more comfortable, more practical and cheaper for them. Such women generally continued to wear Directoire-style knickers which were no longer popular with the fashion-conscious young.

Cami-knickers were popular and these were mostly bias cut as they clung nicely to the body. However, the most popular and fashionable knickers of the time were of French style, made of a light, smooth fabric and bias cut to complement the popular dress styles. These French knickers often had an opening on the side that was secured with a button so no folds would show through and a perfect fit was ensured. Some even had a yoke around the waist (see picture below) to allow a closer fit over the stomach.

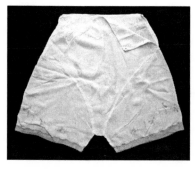

Handmade white rayon French knickers with yoke at the waist and coloured embroidery and net edging around the legs. c.1940. Author's collection.

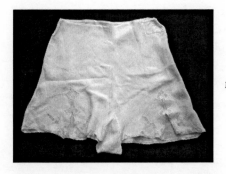

Pink silk machine made French knickers 1930. Author's collection.

Several women remember that, due to the smoothness of French knickers and lack of elastic around the waist and legs, if the button fell off, the knickers could fall to the ground—Iris Massingham experienced this in the early 1940s (see displayed quotation below).

> When I was a teenager in about 1943-44, I was visiting London from Norfolk and at Paddington Station my French knickers fell down to my ankles, as the button had come off! I stepped out of them and put them in my handbag. (1980)
>
> Iris Massingham, Wartime machine worker, born 1923.

> I remember wearing French knickers in 1933 that had a button at the side and lace around the legs. They were a creamy colour in nainsook fabric, a fine cotton muslin. (2009)
>
> Ruby Fisher. Milliner, born 1913.

By the end of the 1930s, all shop-bought knickers were closed at the crotch, although some older women were probably still making their own open styles from old patterns. Ruby Fisher worked in a clothes shop in the 1930s that sold 'fleecy-lined knickers with elastic around the legs and waist; they had an option of long or short legs, but not right up to the hip'. The colours were pink, blue, green and cream.

Towards the end of the decade, the dresses and skirts were shorter and not so tight around the thighs. As the hems were often close to the knee, this meant that some women still preferred knickers of the Directoire style. These were made in rayon, cotton or wool. It was also common for women to hand-knit knickers or cami-knickers for winter wear. Rayon, often referred to as art. silk (artificial silk), had become widely used by this time—the quality of the fabric having improved considerably since the 1920s. Other new fabrics included Sateen: a fine cotton fabric made in the style of satin to give a shine on one side. The 1938 mail-order catalogue of J. D. Williams & Co. Ltd of Manchester offered a large range of knickers, as pictured here.

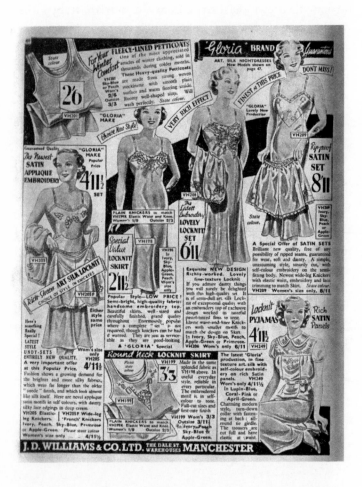

Page from J D Williams catalogue 1938. Courtesy J D Williams.

> I remember that when I wore French
> knickers in the 1940s they made me feel
> elegant. They were quite cool to wear, so I
> only wore them during the summer months.
> (2006)
>
> Mary Charlton, born 1923.

Probably the most fascinating items in the 1938 J. D. Williams catalogue for the costume historian are the 'open-back drawers in two reliable qualities': 'grey fleece-lined drawers' and 'all-wool natural woven drawers'. These were described as 'the old folks' favourite: thick, warm and noted for hard wear; made in roomy sizes, on strong sateen waistbands with tape; full-length legs reaching over the knee with snug-fitting ribbed ends; wrap-over open back'. This advertisement demonstrates that J. D. Williams believed that they had customers who would prefer old-fashioned underwear.

In December 1939, shortly after the outbreak of World War II, the paper pattern company Weldon produced a booklet that included pictures of several types of knickers for which they sold paper patterns. These were mostly in the French style but also showed short-legged knickers with elastic around the waist and legs. However, it also included 'trim, well-cut knickers' without elastic, which they described as 'shorts with a small leg' and 'figure-fitting briefs, darted into the waist'. This design which used minimal fabric and no elastic was rather forward-thinking, as materials for clothing would soon be in short supply.

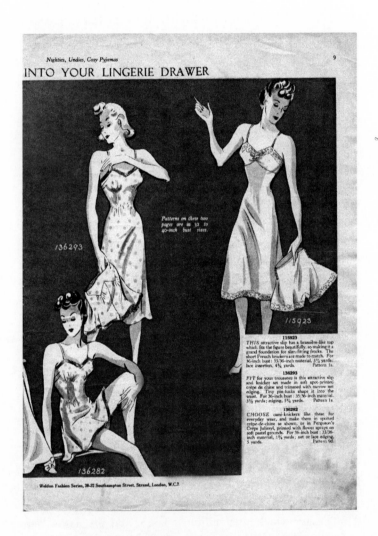

Nighties, Undies, Cosy Pyjamas

INTO YOUR LINGERIE DRAWER

9

Patterns on these two
pages are in 32 to
40-inch bust sizes.

136293

115923

136282

115923
THIS attractive slip has a brassière-like top which fits the figure beautifully, so making it a grand foundation for slim-fitting frocks. The short French knickers are made to match. For 36-inch bust: 35/36-inch material, 3½ yards; lace insertion, 4¾ yards. Pattern 1s.

136293
FIT for your trousseau is this attractive slip and knicker set made in soft spot-printed crêpe de chine and trimmed with narrow net edging. Tiny pin-tucks shape it into the waist. For 36-inch bust : 33/36-inch material, 3½ yards; edging, 5¾ yards. Pattern 1s.

136282
CHOOSE cami-knickers like these for everyday wear, and make them in spotted crêpe-de-chine as shown, or in Ferguson's Crêpe Julienyl, printed with flower sprays on soft pastel grounds. For 36-inch bust : 35/36-inch material, 1⅞ yards; net or lace edging, 5 yards. Pattern 9d.

Weldon Fashion Series, 30-32 Southampton Street, Strand, London, W.C.2.

Pattern from Weldons Fashion Series 1940s

As a result of the war, it was clear that there would be many changes to fashion which would influence the use and styles of underwear. By 1940, it was clear that the British government needed to ration clothing to ensure that all citizens had the opportunity to purchase good, basic items of apparel. Given the demands on cargo space and the risks to merchant shipping from U-boat attacks, it was necessary to severely restrict the import of fabrics and clothing, since imports such as food were obviously more vital. People were encouraged to reduce wastage of fabrics as part of the nation's war effort, and rationing would also help to ensure that people reused fabrics to make smaller items such as knickers.

Clothes rationing began on 1st June 1941. The British Board of Trade provided information on what was to be rationed which was published in several national newspapers. In 1941, women were provided with 66 clothing coupons per year, but by 1943 this was reduced to 48, due to the lack of availability of fabrics. Rationing continued until 1949: four years after the war in Europe had ended.

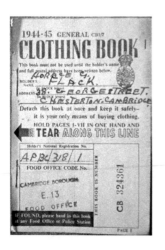

Clothing Ration Book
1944-5. Author's collection

41

Cami-knickers required four coupons, and knickers three. A yard of woollen cloth 36 inches wide needed three coupons, and cotton and other cloth of the same width needed two coupons. Knitting wool needed one coupon for two ounces. Elastic and mending wool and threads were coupon-free, but the lack of restriction sometimes meant that shops were out of stock.

A government initiative known as the Utility Scheme was introduced in Britain in the spring of 1942 in a push to simplify garment styles and thus save on labour and materials. A number of top-grade dress designers worked with the Board of Trade to ensure that the operation was as efficient as possible. All forms of trimming and embroidery were eschewed and gathers and frills avoided in order to use as little fabric as possible. There were strict restrictions relating to the fineness of yarn, closeness of weave, weight of cotton per yard and type of finish. Rayon was the preferred fabric for utility wear and prices were set and controlled by the Board of Trade. (1)

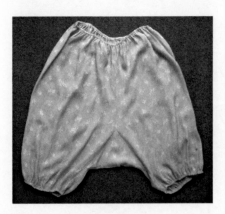

Utility Directoire knickers made from blue rayon with elastic around the waist and legs. c.1945. Author's collection.

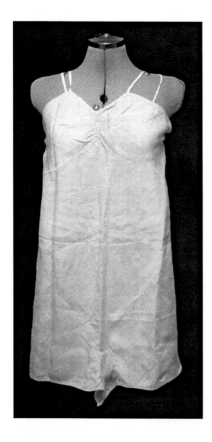

Pink utility
cami-knickers with
plain edging. c.1945.
Author's collection.

Many women have recalled making their own underwear during the war, including knickers made from used fabrics or knitted from damaged woollen garments that they had unpicked. There were many knitting patterns around at this time for several types of knickers. A paperback book entitled *New Clothes from Old* was published in this era which provided patterns and instructions on how to cut and sew clothes from recycled fabrics. The knicker-pattern it offered was of a French style with very wide and open legs and a yoke rather than elastic around the waist (2). The author of the book suggests that this could be cut from the skirt of a damaged dress, and adds 'use buttons and button-holes or button loops for fastening with an opening at the side'. French knickers were very easy to make and to decorate with embroidery or lace.

In September 1943, the *Housewife* magazine noted that 'thin quick-drying lingerie is a possibility in summer—in winter it is an invitation to pneumonia—Don't overlook hand-knitted winter lingerie'. The magazine also suggested that, by this time, there was a serious shortage of materials for making underwear: 'elastic, or rather its disappearance, does raise some problems; pants must now be darted to the waist-line and finished with small buttons and loops'.

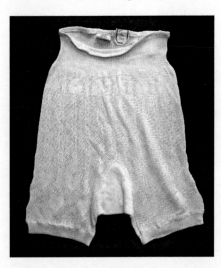

Utility Knickers made from white knitted rayon. These have never been worn because the price label is attached for three shillings and tenpence halfpenny. c.1945. Author's collection.

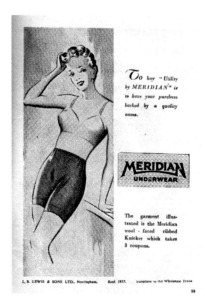

To buy "*Utility* by *MERIDIAN*" is to have your purchase backed by a quality name.

MERIDIAN
UNDERWEAR

The garment illustrated is the Meridian wool - faced ribbed Knicker which takes 3 coupons.

J. B. LEWIS & SONS LTD., Nottingham.   *Regd. 1875.*   Suppliers to the Wholesale Trade

Advertisement from
Housewife Magazine
1944

With wartime restrictions on coal, homes were often quite cold, as were air raid shelters, so cosy knickers and underwear were, naturally, considered a necessity. Many civilian women spent time fire-watching during the Blitz looking out for incendiary bombs and helping to extinguish fires. A fair number of women also worked in the Women's Land Army, helping farmers to grow food. Both of these pursuits exposed women to cold weather and necessitated the wearing of warm underwear.

> When I was in the Land Army during the war, I remember that the Government provided outside clothing, but not underwear. I had to buy my own underwear which consisted of using my coupons. (2010)
>
> Irene Bunn, born 1924.

Women in the services wore plain and utilitarian knickers with ribbed or elasticated legs and waist which would help keep out the cold. (Ribbing is vertical lines of knitted fabric.) The knickers were usually made of wool or cotton in colours to complement their military uniforms which were cream, pale khaki or navy blue.

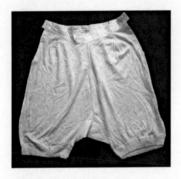

Cream coloured Woman's
Army knickers 1943.
Author's collection.

At the end of World War II in 1945, Mary Charlton, a member of the Women's Forces, was stationed in Italy where she was able to purchase some beautiful pure-silk lingerie, including cami-knickers, of a quality that would have been impossible to find in Britain then. Mary said that there appeared to be no clothes rationing in Italy at that time.

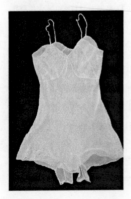

Very fine white silk cami knickers
purchased in Italy 1945. Courtesy
Mary Charlton

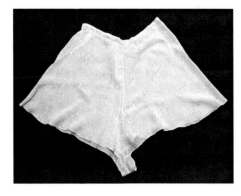

Trousseau 1948.
Hand made pink
silk. Courtesy
Mary Charlton

During the war, women had largely been deprived of clothing made from delicate fabrics for reasons of scarcity and practicality. So as the war came to an end, women were keen to have access to feminine clothing again. Nylon was a new and exciting fabric that most British women had heard about but only a few had come across in the war years (e.g. in gifts of nylon stockings from US soldiers). Nylon did not shrink, it was not susceptible to mildew and it was a strong fabric with colours that did not fade or run. It was also moth-proof, non-iron and very easy to wash and dry. All these assets were very important at the time. However, it was not until the early 1950s that nylon lingerie was very available in British shops.

Nylon was first launched by the American company Du Pont in 1938 and the first nylon stockings were sold in the USA. After America's entry into the war in December 1941, the Du Pont Company was commandeered by the US War Production Board to make parachutes, and ropes and this interrupted their progress in designing fashion clothing. Parachutes that were no longer airworthy were sold to the public so that they could use the fabric. At the beginning of the war parachutes were made of silk, but later they were made of nylon and both provided a wonderful recycling fabric for making pretty and feminine underwear, including knickers.

Du Pont licensed some other companies to produce nylon yarn around the world, including Courtaulds and ICI (Imperial Chemical Industries) in Britain who took on a licence jointly in 1940, founding a new company which they called British Nylon Spinners. It was not until 1958 that the company renamed its product Bri-Nylon: a shortened version of British Nylon.(3)

It is widely believed that Nylon was named after New York and London, the two cities in which it was supposedly discovered simultaneously, but this is entirely without foundation. It was clearly impractical for Du Pont to market their new fabric as 'hexadecamethylene dicarboxylic', so it was initially christened 'Rayon 6-6'. The company soon realised that this risked confusion with the cellulose fabric 'rayon' and changed the working name to the distinctly lacklustre 'Fiber 66' and began to cast around for an enduring alternative that would be original, simple and catchy. Of the several hundred ideas that were considered, Dr Earnest K. Gladding, the soon-to-be manager of Du Pont's nylon division, favoured 'norun', but after tests demonstrated that in fact the product *did* run he was forced to think again. Gladding found himself playing around with anagrams of 'norun' and came up with 'nuron', although this sounded far too much like the word 'neuron', so the 'u' was changed to an 'i', the 'i' to a 'y', and the ultimately meaningless name Nylon was finally born.(4)

The decades following the war would see an explosion in choice, colour and style of all types of clothing, including underwear, as younger women tried hard to separate themselves from previous generations which they regarded as blighted by hardship and horror.

Chapter 4 references

1   Wilson E and Taylor J, *Through the Looking Glass*, BBC Books, 1989, p.118
2   Franks C, *New Clothes from Old*, Evans Brothers Ltd, (c. 1943)
3   Handley S, *Nylon: The Manmade Fashion Revolution*, Bloomsbury Publishing plc, 1999
4   Handley S, *Nylon: The Manmade Fashion Revolution*, Bloomsbury Publishing plc, 1999

Chapter 5

AUSTERITY TO AFFLUENCE

1946–2010

The 'New Look' with longer and fuller skirts was created by French designer Christian Dior in 1947, but not introduced into Britain until 1948. While rationing continued, this new fashion would have used many coupons because of the quantity of fabric used. When rationing ended, the New Look was still unavailable to most ordinary women but was being worn by the younger members of the Royal Family and other wealthy people. Some of the *couturier* styles at the time (from top-grade French dress designers) consisted of rather tight skirts, so these needed tight-fitting underwear for which French knickers and cami-knickers continued to be popular.

During the 1950s, nylon became a very important and popular fabric which was used in factories to mass produce underwear. Nylon knickers were easy to wash and dry. They were becoming smaller and were now referred to as briefs. Nylon knickers were often very pretty with nylon embroidery and lace around the legs and in many soft and pretty colours.

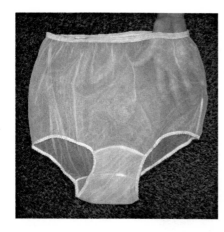

Pale blue sheer nylon
knickers c.1955.
Author's collection.

My mother-in-law hand stitched her
own French style knickers in the 1950s
and always made her own knickers up
to her death in 1976. (2009)

Phyllis Dyke. Born 1925

Sheer nylon knickers were being sold in the late 1950s. They
were flimsy and very see through. This was an exciting new
fabric and made many young women feel feminine. It was
certainly competitive with silk underwear.

In the book 'The New Fibers' 1946, the writers state that 'nylon
is still quite expensive, although substantial price reductions
have been made and undoubtedly will continue in the future.'
(1) They also note results from a 'toughness index' where it

was found that nylon was more than twice as tough as rayon at the time and that the toughness of silk was in between the two.

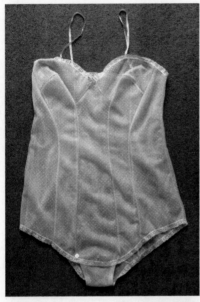

Pale mauve sheer nylon cami-knickers 1950s. Author's collection.

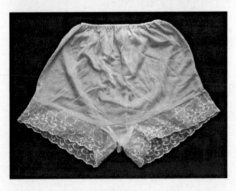

Pale blue nylon knickers edged with coloured nylon embroidered lace. c. 1958. Author's collection

However, the wearing of nylon knickers did not remain highly popular for many people as they did not absorb moisture, so were not comfortable in hot weather as they could cause irritation to the skin.

It was several years before the Second World War stopped having an effect on fashion and textiles due to rationing which continued until 1949 and Utility which continued until 1952

During the 1950s glamour was very important due to women having been deprived for so long due to the war and its lasting effects into the early 1950s. It was a very shapely and feminine decade where women were returning to their former roles. It was also a time where the housewife was seen as an important asset to the family and women's magazines at the time boosted their role, often suggesting that they needed to do look after themselves in a way that would please their husbands, such as wearing pretty clothes which must have included underwear. Knickers were now no longer a taboo subject and in 1957 Marilyn Monroe stood over an air vent which raised her skirt and showed her knickers in the film 'The Seven Year Itch.' It is clear that they were pretty and fitted snugly around her waist and legs.

The American Burlesque entertainment show in the 1930s mainly consisted of striptease artists, some wearing and removing 'G' string knickers which were of a small triangular style tied together at the sides with tape. In the 1950s this fashion caught on for beach bikinis.

Lycra was a synthetic man-made elastic fibre invented in the USA by DuPont in the late 1950s. At first it was used for sports and swimwear, but towards the end of the 20th century, it ensured a really good and comfortable fit for knickers.

At the end of the 1950s lycra allowed underwear to be stretchy in both directions and very comfortable to wear. This was mostly used for pantie girdles which were worn by young women who were pleased to avoid the previously heavyweight corsets worn by previous generations. Pantie girdles were a lightweight corset style of knickers that held the tummy in and were edged with a suspender on each side front and back to hold up stockings.

The fashion for camiknickers was slowly declining over the years, probably because they had been worn by the mothers of the new generation who viewed them as old fashioned.

Black underwear was now much more popular, although some women still saw it as sexy, but not terribly erotic any more. Sheer nylon in black was pretty and feminine and different styles of knickers were made in this fabric.

> When my elderly aunt (born 1887) died in 1968
> I cleared out her house and found a pair of light
> tweed directorie knickers, which she probably
> wore for working on her smallholding during the
> colder months. (2009)
>
> Phyllis Dyke. Born 1925

The 1960s was a decade of huge changes in fashion mainly because of the post-war baby boom becoming teenagers, and the fact that full employment early in the decade provided them with money to spend on fashions.

Due to the slim and straight fitting styles from the early 1960s many more women now wore panty girdles.

In the early 1960s a fashion developed that was known as 'hipster' skirts and trousers. The hipster style meant that they were below the waist and held around the upper thighs. This was a fashion for teenage girls only. Due to this fashion, ordinary knickers would have shown around the waist, so hipster knickers became available and in fact they have remained so until modern times.

> I remember when nylon knickers were introduced; we were able to wear clean knickers every day. (2009)
>
> Rochelle Mortimer-Massingham born 1945. Museum Worker

A fabric known as 'stretch nylon' was available from the mid 1960s. Stretch nylon knickers were comfortable to wear as they stretched nicely over the hips and allowed much more freedom of movement. Another new design for this fabric was the body stocking which was similar to cami-knickers, but much more tight fitting and stretchy. This was a boom time for all synthetic fabrics as the technology was improving all the time and many people were very pleased to try out the new fabrics.

In the book 'I Haven't a Thing to Wear' (1965), Liane Keene provided a list 'For the basic underwear wardrobe.' She suggested '3 pairs of briefs . . . 3 slip and pantie sets OR 3 pairs of cami-knickers. She described cami-knickers as 'blissfully comfortable, especially under suits.' She wrote 'Don't try to save elastic by avoiding smalls washing' and that elastic should be replaced when it is no longer doing the job it should. Women from that generation recall that they would not have worn cami-knickers as they were viewed as old fashioned. No-one remembered them being sold in shops at that time.

> When I was a district nurse in the early 1960s, I was giving an elderly lady a blanket bath in her own home. The home help came into the room with the clothes to dress her. They consisted of open crotch drawers of an Edwardian style. The home help told me that these drawers were known as 'Ready Boys.'
> (2008)
>
> Phyllis Dyke born 1925

During the same decade disposable paper knickers were on sale and people often took them on holiday. They were quite cheap and wore very well for a whole day. By the mid 1970s they were no longer available.

As usual, directoires were still available for older women, but they now could be made of nylon which made laundering much easier. However, many older women were continuing to wear them made from woollen or cotton knitted fabrics.

Due to the very short skirts in 1967, tights became a fashion that was happily adopted by all young women. A bride in 1968 remembered wearing torquoise stretch nylon knickers with stockings attached. They were called 'pantie hose.' For her trousseau she recalled buying two bra-petticoats with matching hipster knickers. One set was a turquoise patterned nylon fabric and the other was in an orange patterned fabric, two colours that were highly fashionable at the time.

During the 1970s many fabrics were available that consisted of mixed fibres including nylon which made them hard wearing and easy to launder. These were popular because they were more absorbent than pure nylon underwear which often caused a sweat rash.

The 1970s saw the introduction of a large range of knicker styles, many of them similar to those of much earlier times. Some knickers were of a bikini style and very small, while others had tight legs that went halfway down the thigh, possibly for use under trousers. There was also a very brief style of panties with an elasticated waistband. These consisted of a triangle of fabric at the front and back that were held together with a thin line of elastic over the hips. This style was very similar to the earlier 'G'strings.

Moulded underwear became available from the 1970s and has remained so ever since. This was a new technique where thermoplastic fabrics were moulded into shape by heating.

Aerobics and gymnastics were popular pastimes in the 1980s and due to the tight and clinging fabrics that had Lycra blended with them, it became fashionable to wear these costumes with very long leg openings with came right up to the hip. This made the legs look much longer than they were. A range of knickers was then produced following this style known as 'high leg' knickers.

Cami-knickers, now known as a 'Teddy' (originally an American term) were very similar to those worn 50 years earlier and many were made of pure silk. French knickers were reintroduced and worn by young women, possibly very popular as trousseau underwear.

In 1992 fashion designer Vivien Westwood attended a function at Buckingham Palace. On the way out she spun around allowing her skirt to rise to her waist. This showed that she was not wearing any form of knickers, only tights.

Thongs were introduced in the late 1990s and were extremely popular for young women to wear with tight skirts or trousers. It became acceptable that when they bent over, the top of the thongs could be seen above the trouser line.

> I wear thongs under tight trousers, but other styles of knickers have become available which do not show under tight clothes. I would not wear thongs for long journeys—they cut you in half! (2009)
>
> Theresa Coyne born 1949

Open crotch knickers have been available in sex shops for many years, but have not been acceptable for regular wear. Rather interestingly, they are now being recommended for use by disabled people or those with an incontinence problem. In

2006 the Disabled Living Foundation produced a Factsheet for incontinence sufferers which stated 'crotchless knickers may be bought from adult shops/mail order catalogues.' In 2004 the Muscular Dystrophy Foundation also recommended the use of crotchless knickers for use by wheelchair users making it easier for them to use the toilet.

It seems that the future will have no very new ideas on knicker wear, but just use the older styles in a more fashionable modern way.

When I was a young mother I remember putting elastic into knickers where the elastic had broken. (2009)

Rochellle Mortimer-Massingham. Born 1945
Museum Worker

Chapter 5 references

1. Sherman J V & Sherman S. The New Fibres: With a Classified List of Patents 1946 p.36
2. Liame Keen. I haven't a Thing to Wear. P.39

Appendix 1

TIME LINE

1795 first wearing of long legged tight pantaloons

1810 drawers now worn which consisted of two legs drawn together at the waist with an open crotch

1820 drawers became shorter ending just below the knee

1830s drawers no longer a fashion item

1840s drawers returned to fashion

1850s now longer legged and much more elaborately made

1860 the word bloomers now sometimes used

1860s drawers now worn by middle class women

1860s knickerbockers introduced

1870s drawers now had shorter legs and some had a closed crotch

1880s working class women began to wear open crotch drawers

1880s the fabric Aertex used

1880s combinations introduced

1900s drawers now very frilly

1910 closed crotch now more widely available

1906 French drawers introduced, very wide and to the knees with frills

1908 Directoire knickers first worn

1914 Peg Top knickers fashionable for a short time

1915 Closed crotch now often worn by working class women

1917 Chemi knickers introduced
1920s Cami knickers became fashionable
1924 Small knickers became known as panties
1928 Trinity Set worn by young women
1930 No open crotch knickers available in shops
1930 Small knickers now called trunks
1930s Much smaller and shorter French knickers
1930s Rayon now used frequently
1950 Nylon now used for some knickers
Late 1950s Lycra invented by DuPont
Early 1960s Hipster knickers fashionable
Mid 1960s Stretch nylon knickers available
1973 Paper disposable knickers sold
1970s Moulded underwear now used
1980s High leg knickers very commonly used
Late 1990s Thongs became fashionable

Appendix 2

COLLECTING DRAWERS AND

KNICKERS

The collecting of vintage underwear is a fascinating and rewarding pastime, which offers real scope for original research. Collectable items are relatively plentiful, and often do not command high prices. Drawers from the 19th century can still be found in junk shops or old clothes shops, but they are often stained and torn. Knickers from the 1930s and 40s are easier to find, and are often in better condition. The ones that have usually survived are made of cotton, or rayon. If they are silk, they are often damaged. Old silk has sometimes been treated with metal compounds to make the fabric heavier. This does not do well over time and the fibre often breaks down. This is known as 'shattered silk.' Also, some shopkeepers try to clean them up using biological detergents which ruin them as the chemicals are meant to digest protein and silk is pure protein.

It is not a good idea to use chlorine bleach to remove stains from old clothes as it will help to diminish the old fibres. There is a gentle bleach made form plant materials which works well without damaging the items. Old underwear sometimes has small rust-like stains which are not possible to remove with any bleaching agent. These stains are usually from iron in the water in which they have been washed.

Damaged drawers and knickers can sometimes be repaired as long as it does not change the original style. Dirty marks are often easy to remove from cotton drawers just by washing them carefully in a non biological detergent. If I need to wash silk items, I squeeze them through in warm water with a washing product especially made for silk and delicate fabrics. I think we have to accept that some stains on all old clothes are not possible to remove without causing damage to the fabric. Starch should never be used on old clothing as it can cause tears and other damage.

Old clothing must be ironed carefully with an iron that is not too hot. This works best if the garment is not totally dry. Silk is best ironed with a cool iron while damp.

I catalogue my collection by numbering the items and putting the details onto an Excel computer file. I cut out small squares of cotton, or linen fabric and write the number onto it in pencil. I then sew the number inside the item with a couple of hand stitches. When entering the details into the catalogue, I note the type of fabric and fasteners and whether it is hand or machine made. I also note the provenance if it is known. I think it is also important to note what could be original repairs and what repairs you might have done for their conservation.

If anything old needs to be repaired, it is best to use pure cotton thread, or pure silk for silk underwear. I only repair tears if they are vulnerable to becoming worse. I have a collection of old buttons that I am sometimes able to use if a button is missing, but that is always noted in my costume catalogue. I also have a collection of old white cotton tape which I have found at car boot sales and junk shops and it is often useful for repairing or replacing those that are worn, or broken.

I do not display my costume collection, because I believe old items of underwear wear should be conserved and protected from damage by light or dust. The garments are gently rolled, rather than folded. They are stored in plastic containers with lids. Containers should then be stored in a dark and dry area of the house.

INDEX

Aertex, 16, 17, 61

Angola cotton, 9

Army and Navy Stores, 22

Bible, 5

Bikini style, 57

Bloomers, 4, 11, 28, 61

Briefs, 2, 4, 39, 50, 56

Bri nylon, 48

Broderie Anglaise, 10, 14

Butterick, 12, 21, 26

Calico, 9, 13, 15, 19, 22

Cami bockers, 29

Cami knickers, 27-29, 32, 35, 37, 42, 43, 46, 50, 52, 55, 56, 58, 62

Chamois leather, 9

Chemi knickers, 27, 62

Closed crotch style, 4, 5, 13, 18-20, 22-24, 26, 28, 61

Combinations, 13-17, 21, 27, 29, 61

Cotton stocking web, 9

Crepe de Chine, 28

Crinoline, 9, 10, 12, 13

De Medici Catherine, 3

Depression The, 34

Directoire, 22, 23, 28, 29, 32, 35, 37, 42, 56, 61

Disposable knickers, 56, 62

Drawers, 1, 3-7, 9, 10-13, 14-16, 19-22, 26, 28, 39, 56, 61

Duchess of Argyle, 28

Duchess of Kent, 6

DuPont, 53, 62

Feather stitching, 14, 15, 22

First World War, 26

Flannel, 9, 11, 12, 19

Fleecy lined knickers, 37

French knickers, 28, 29, 31, 32, 35, 36, 39, 44, 50, 58, 62

Gamages, 23, 24, 26

G strings, 57

High leg, 58, 62

Hipsters, 55

ICI, 48

Jaeger Dr Gustav, 16

Knickerbockers, 21, 22, 24, 61

Knickers, 4, 13, 16, 18, 22-27

Knitted knickers, 43, 44

Lady Chesterfield, 19

Lady Stanley, 6

Lancet The 15

Lingerie, 19, 28, 29, 44, 46, 47

Longcloth, 9, 13, 25

Lycra, 53, 54, 57, 62

Joan of Arc, 5

Madeira Embroidery, 20

Maillot Jean Christophe, 5

Marilyn Monroe, 53

Moulded underwear, 57, 62

Muslin Dresses, 4, 6

Nainsook, 21, 25, 36

New woman, 20

New Look, 50

Nylon, 4, 47, 48, 50-52, 54-57, 62

Pantaloons, 4-6, 51

Pantie Girdles, 54

Pantie Hose, 57

Panties, 4, 57, 62

Peg top knickers, 25, 26

Pepys Samuel, 3

Prince Albert, 12

Princess Charlotte, 6

Rational Dress Society, 16

Rationing, 41, 46, 50, 53

Rayon, 4, 31, 32, 35, 37, 42, 44, 48, 52, 62

Ribbon trimming, 20

Sartor manufacturing, 29

Sateen, 25, 37, 39

Second World War, 53

Shattered silk, 63

Sheer nylon, 51, 52, 54

Stockinette, 16

Stretch nylon, 55, 57, 62

Tango knickers, 24

Teddy, 58

Thongs, 58, 62

Trunks, 4, 62

Tucks, 10, 11

Undies, 29

Utility Scheme, 42

Washing and ironing, 64

Women's Land Army, 45

Lightning Source UK Ltd.
Milton Keynes UK
UKOW051908240112

185985UK00001B/18/P